DESKTOP

CYCLING CLASS

Illustrated by

Rami Niemi

T0364025

RP Minis®
Hachette Book Group
1290 Avenue of the Americas, New York, NY 10104
www.runningpress.com
@Running_Press

First Edition: April 2023

Published by RP Minis, an imprint of Perseus Books, LLC,
a subsidiary of Hachette Book Group, Inc. The RP Minis
name and logo is a registered trademark of the Hachette
Book Group.

The publisher is not responsible for websites (or their
content) that are not owned by the publisher.

ISBN: 978-0-7624-8215-3

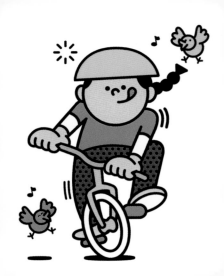

INTRODUCTION

If you know how to ride a bike, your earliest cycling experiences were likely full of trial and error (not to mention the occasional scrape and bruise). First you used training wheels. Then you graduated to pumping your feet while someone ran behind you holding your seat upright. And eventually you found your balance. You learned to steer. It all

came together, and you sailed trium-
phantly down the sidewalk, your hair
blowing in the wind (under a sensible
helmet, of course).

Riding a bike is exhilarating! And
it's excellent exercise. But carving out
time to get in a ride can be tough. Plus
there's the weather to consider—rain,
extreme heat, snow, hail, fog, and
strong winds are not conducive to
comfortable riding. That's where the

Desktop Cycling Class comes in handy. Get in a workout without leaving the comfort of your office? Yes please!

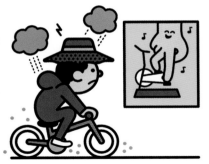

Inside this kit you'll find every-thing you need to hold your very own Desktop Cycling Class. Take a look at the diagram and get familiar with the bike before you begin.

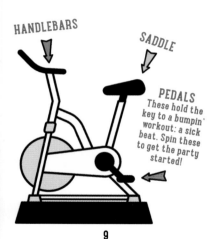

HANDLEBARS

SADDLE

PEDALS
These hold the key to a bumpin' workout: a sick beat. Spin these to get the party started!

9

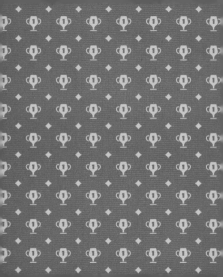

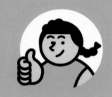

Safety First

A note on safety: Desktop cycling may sound like simple fun, but as with any type of exercise, safety and success go hand in hand. Here are some pointers:

1. **Please refrain from riding with only one finger. You can't count on just one finger to do all the work. This is a joint effort.**

2. **Keep your fingers on the pedals and OFF the handlebars. That kind of showy behavior can only lead to trouble. Does it look cool? Sure.**

Does that mean you should do it?
Depends on who's watching.

3. If you're feeling dizzy, slow down
   or take a break. You don't have to
   work your fingers to the bone to
   reap the benefits of the Desktop
   Cycling Class.

4. Lastly, it's important to stay
   hydrated. Drink water before your
   workout and remember to keep a
   bottle handy.

Let's talk about **strength**, **power**, and **endurance**. These are all key components of a good workout. In the Desktop Cycling Class, you will utilize and build all three skills. With time and practice, you'll see improvements in all areas, both on and off the bike.

Strength is what you use when your muscles push back against resistance. The stronger you are, the more resistance you can endure.

Strength can be measured by the amount of weight you're able to successfully lift. You use your strength when completing exercises in a slow and controlled manner. Pedaling up a steep hill uses strength.

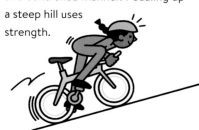

Power is your ability to move weight *with speed*. When you're pushing on the pedals trying to go faster, you're using your power. A good example is a runner waiting to start a race. That first moment after the starting pistol sounds, a runner uses explosive force to propel themselves forward. Power is strength and speed working together.

Endurance is about keeping yourself pushing for a long period of time. Marathon runners need to have a great deal of endurance to be able to run for so long. The more you ride, the more endurance you will build. And there's no better time to start than right now!

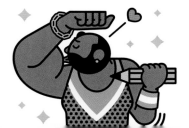

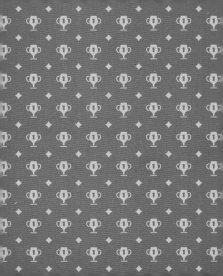

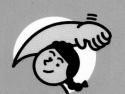

Warm It Up

The following pages will walk you through some warmup exercises designed to get your fingers ready to work. It's important to prepare yourself properly, both physically and mentally. Start by taking a look at your workout space. If you've been avoiding straightening up your desk, now is the time to do it. Clear away the stray paperclips, old cups of coffee, and stacks of papers.

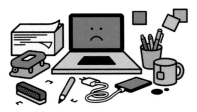

Now that your physical space is ready, take a moment to clear the clutter from your mind. Put aside any worries to make room for this act of self-care. You're so accustomed to having your hands full, it may take some time to let go of any tension from your day. Close your eyes and take a few deep breaths.

Remove any tight rings or watches. Make sure you're comfortable and able to move freely. When you feel ready, turn the page and kick things off!

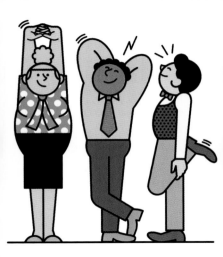

The warmup begins with stretches. Hold your hand in an upside down "peace" sign, fingers resting on the desk. Bending your fingers, alternate raising your pointer and middle fingers like you're lifting their "knees." Let's see you lengthen those ligaments!

Next, see how high you can stretch each finger. Keeping your finger straight, raise it as high as it can comfortably go. Keep the other finger on the desk, then alternate. Hold each stretch for a count of 10. You should be starting to feel loose!

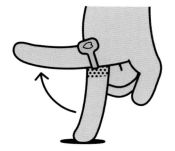

Next, let's get your appendages familiar with the proper form. Pick your hand up off the desk. Keeping it upright, fingers pointing down, alternate reaching your pointer and middle fingers as if you're bicycling them in the air. Imagine with each stroke that you're pushing on pedals. Your fingertips should be tracing circles in the air. Start slowly and build to your quickest pace, making sure not to lose your form. Keep it up for 30 seconds!

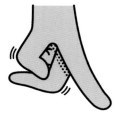

Feeling more warmed up? Your knuckles will thank you later!

Next, let's practice jumps. Start with straight fingers on the desk, in the "peace" position. Working

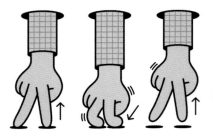

together, bend both fingers and press down with your fingertips. Launch your hand up into the air, then return to the starting position. Repeat the jump 10 times.

You should now be feeling all warmed up and excited for the main event. Grab a sip of water and a towel. Get ready to get your hand(s) dirty!

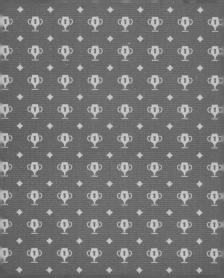

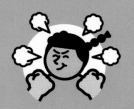

Feel the Burn

Your joints are loose and your tendons are warmed up. You're about to experience the ride of your life. It's time to hustle for that muscle!

The next few pages will walk you through the key positions of the Desktop Cycling Class. It's up to you how long you stay in each one. Try each position for a minute. Then try cycling through the positions until you've done each three times. Listen to your body and do what feels right. And don't forget to cool down at the end of your workout!

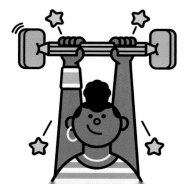

Seated Position

You begin your workout in seated position. Rest on the saddle with your fingertips touching the pedals. Get spinning to start the music! Feel the rhythm and begin to pump your fingers to the beat. You've got this!

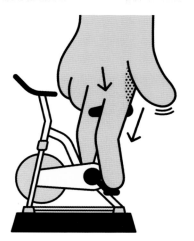

35

Standing Position

Next, you move to standing position. With your fingertips on the pedals, push away from the saddle, keeping your fingers straight. Without sitting back down, start to pedal away. Now your muscles are really working. It should feel like you're biking up a hill. Keep pumping those pedals!

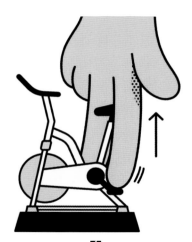

37

Standing Jumps

Last but not least: You've made it to standing jumps. Give yourself a pat on the back—you're almost done! Here, you keep pedaling your fingers while you lift on and off the saddle. Move up and down to the beat of the music. It may take some time to get the rhythm right, but keep at it. Work those tendons!

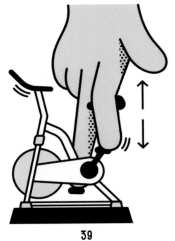

39

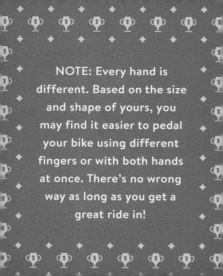

NOTE: Every hand is different. Based on the size and shape of yours, you may find it easier to pedal your bike using different fingers or with both hands at once. There's no wrong way as long as you get a great ride in!

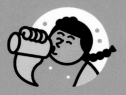

Cool Down

Just as warming up gets your body ready to move, cooling down prepares your body to go back to its resting state. Your heart rate is elevated during a workout, and you want to lower it gradually. If you stop exercising suddenly and your heart rate drops, you may feel a bit dizzy or woozy. But you can prevent that with a gentle cool down.

Try walking or marching your fingers in place while focusing on breathing deeply. Stretching your muscles is another great cool-down exercise and also helps to improve overall flexibility.

Give yourself a hand—you have completed the Desktop Cycling Class!

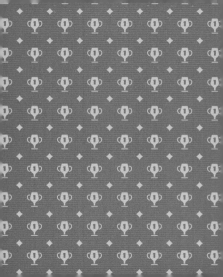

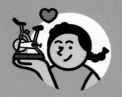

Keep It Going

You've got to hand it to yourself: You did an awesome job! You're off to a great start, but one Desktop Cycling Class isn't going to keep you fit forever. Working exercise into your schedule is the next hurdle. There will be times you feel busy or tired and don't want to lift a finger. On those days, you must tell yourself there will be no excuses or finger-pointing. And if some days are harder than others, that's perfectly normal. Remember, it's the ride, not the destination, that counts!

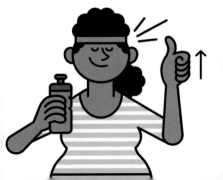

This book has been bound
using handcraft methods and
Smyth-sewn to ensure durability.

The dust jacket and interior were
illustrated by Rami Niemi
and designed by Rachel Peckman.

The text was written
by Eliza Berkowitz.